HEALTH AND MEDICINE

JENNY BRYAN

Wayland

CONTENTS

First published in 1996 by
Wayland (Publishers) Limited
61 Western Road, Hove, East
Sussex BN3 1JD, England
© Copyright 1996 Wayland
(Publishers) Ltd

British Library Cataloguing in
Publication Data
Bryan, Jenny
Health and Medicine. (Science
Discovery Series)
I. Title II. Series
613

ISBN 0 7502 1237 3

Acknowledgements
This book was prepared for
Wayland (Publishers) Limited by
Globe Education
of Nantwich, Cheshire

Concept David Jefferis
Illustrations Peter Bull
Printed and bound by G. Canale
and C.S.p.A., Turin

Picture Credits
Art Directors 27
Image Select 9l, 9r
Life File 29b, 31
Popperfoto 15, 24, 29t, 43, 46, 47
Science Photo Library *Front cover* (bl,
c, tr, br), 4, 6t, 8l, 8r, 10, 11, 12-13, 14,
16, 17, 18, 19, 20l, 20r, 21, 22, 22-23,
24l, 25, 26l, 26r, 27, 28, 30, 32-33, 33,
34, 35, 36, 37, 38, 39, 40, 41, 42, 45
Tony Stone *Back cover* 5, 6b
Topham 7l, 7r, 14b

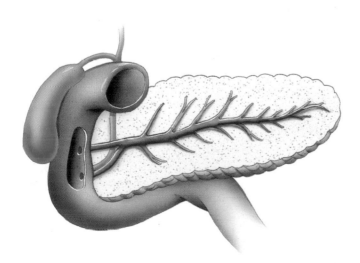

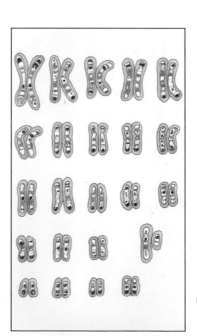

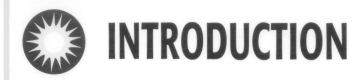

INTRODUCTION

For thousands of years medical research has had one overriding goal – to help us live longer. Early discoveries about how the body works laid the foundations for more recent advances in preventing and curing disease.

Making a discovery in medicine is only the beginning. It can take years for scientists to get their work accepted. Medical research is a long, hard business. But for those who succeed there is the reward of knowing that they have improved the way we live.

▼ Scientists knew a defective gene was responsible for many cases of inherited breast cancer, but the research required to find where that gene was located in human DNA, was painstakingly slow.

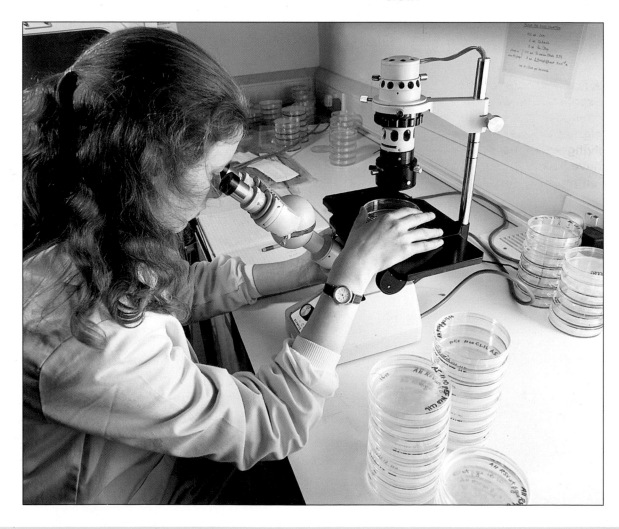

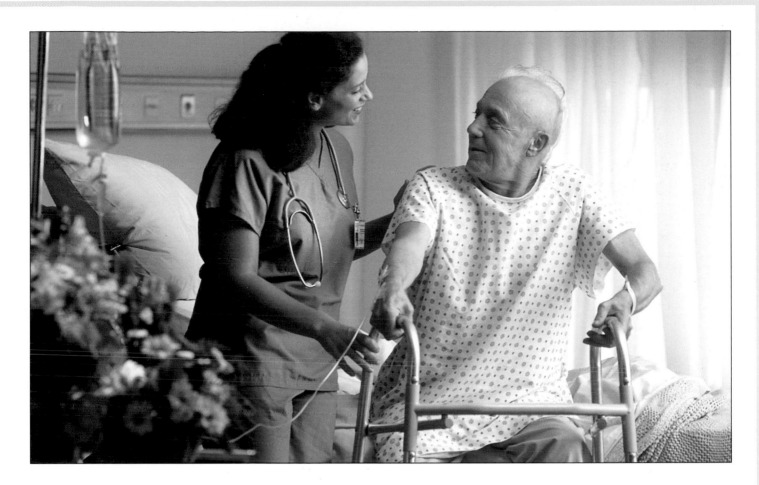

▲ Many people today can expect to live well into their seventies and even their eighties. Better standards of living and better health care have both contributed to longer lifetimes.

Until the start of the twentieth century, only a few men and women lived to celebrate their fortieth birthday. Most died young from infection or poor nutrition. Today, people living in industrialized places, like America, Europe, Australasia and Japan, can expect to live well into their seventies. Better hygiene, vaccination and new treatments for many killer diseases have all helped to improve life for these people.

The same is not true for people living in the developing areas of the world – Africa, South America and many parts of Asia. Only a small amount of medical research has been aimed at treating their health problems, such as poor diet, malaria, and other tropical infections. Developing countries do not have the money to pay for their own research programmes, and they cannot afford the expensive drugs and equipment that are available to treat the health problems endured by many of their people.

MEDICAL ETHICS

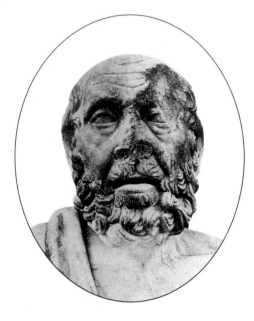

▲ Hippocrates travelled widely, visited Egypt and founded a school of medicine on the island of Kos in Greece. This sculpture is from Ostia in Italy and is Roman.

▶ Patients under anaesthetic need to have confidence that the surgeon will perform the right operation. If it is your heart that needs attention you do not want to wake up to find your leg amputated.

From earliest times, doctors have made a promise when they finish their training and pass all their exams. The most important part of that promise is that they will treat their patients to the very best of their ability and will never deliberately harm anyone. The original promise that doctors made was called the Hippocratic Oath. It was named after Hippocrates, a Greek doctor believed to have lived between 460 and 370 BC. The oath is one of sixty medical writings called the Hippocratic Collection, which Hippocrates and his followers are thought to have written. The exact words of the promise have changed over the centuries and religion has also played a part, but whatever a doctor's religion, he or she undertakes always to put the needs of the patient above everything else.

Hippocrates is credited with the first medical teaching that had a scientific basis. He examined his patients and watched what happened to them. He wrote down what he saw and linked different findings together. His ideas about disease were not correct but he laid the foundations for the way modern medicine is practised. Above all, he put his patients first.

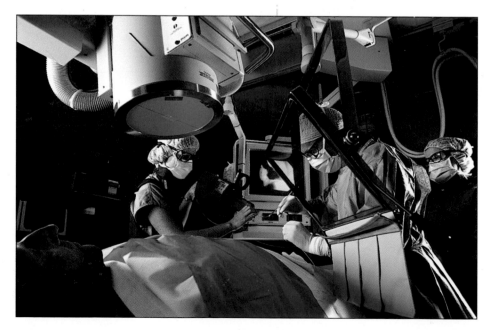

JOSEF MENGELE

Josef Mengele was probably the most evil doctor who ever lived. He certainly did not keep his promise as a doctor not to harm patients. He was the doctor at Auschwitz concentration camp in Poland during the Second World War (1939–1945), and he is held responsible for the deaths of 400,000 people, mostly Jews, in horrific medical experiments. None of his patients willingly consented to the tests they took part in.

After the war, he should have been put on trial for murder. But he escaped and is believed to have lived in South America, probably until the late 1970s. In 1985, a body found in Brazil was identified as that of the notorious Josef Mengele.

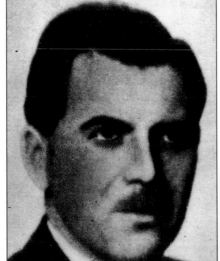

◄ Josef Mengele, the notorious doctor whose medical experiments caused the death of many of the inmates of Auschwitz concentration camp during the Second World War.

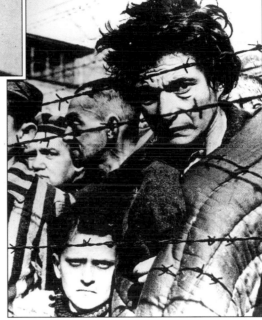

▶ The haggard faces of some of those at Auschwitz who survived long enough to be liberated in 1945 when the war ended.

The oath that doctors take has had a huge effect on the way that medical research is carried out and the way that discoveries are made. If you need to find out the composition of a rock, you can smash it into little pieces and examine the bits. You cannot cut open a healthy living human being just to find out why it works.

If you want to test a new electrical system, you can connect it up, and watch what happens. But you cannot just give an experimental drug to people, even if they are ill, in case it makes them worse. You must test the drug thoroughly before giving it because the patient's safety must come first.

Before any human takes part in a medical experiment the doctor should seek his or her permission. The researcher should explain exactly what will happen. The patient must understand the likely benefits and risks of what is planned. The experiment should only go ahead if the patient is completely happy about taking part. If the patient says 'no', the decision should be final. It may slow down the research but that does not matter.

ANATOMY

natomy is the study of the structure of living organisms. Without it, none of the great medical discoveries would have been possible. Over 3,000 years ago, ancient Egyptians knew the layout of the inside of the human body because they took out nearly all of a dead person's organs before the body was preserved with chemicals, ready for burial. But they left behind few reports of their discoveries.

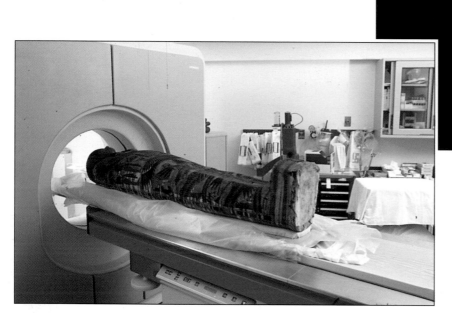

◄ An Egyptian mummy in its painted coffin is investigated using a body scanner. This device enables scientists to discover the condition of the body without needing to disturb the contents of the coffin.

round 300 BC, when Egypt was under Greek rule, scholars in Alexandria, on the Mediterranean coast of Egypt started to cut up bodies in order to study them. They used mainly the bodies of criminals and studied the heart, the brain and other parts. With the spread of Christianity, people began to think dissection of humans was degrading, so researchers had to cut up animals instead.

One of these researchers was a physician called Galen who lived from about AD 130–200. His writings formed the basis of medicine for hundreds of years, but although his work was very useful, he got a lot wrong. For example, he thought that food was absorbed and converted into blood in the liver, where it was filled with natural spirits.

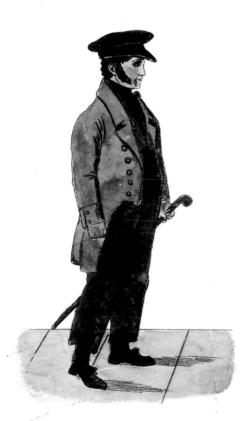

◀ The muscles of the human body are shown in this false-colour copy of an engraving, which originally appeared in *De Humani Corporis Fabrica* by Andreas Vesalius, first published in 1543.

Many of the anatomical diagrams of the thirteenth to fifteenth centuries were more artistic than accurate. However, the Italian artist, Leonardo da Vinci (1452–1519), made drawings based on dissection. He not only made accurate anatomical drawings, he also conveyed something of how bones and muscles worked together to allow movement.

A big leap forward happened when a young Belgian named Andreas Vesalius (1514–1564) started to perform dissections openly in Padua, Italy. He published volume after volume of drawings of the inside of the human body. In detailed pictures, he peeled back layer after layer of skin, muscle and connective tissues to reveal the organs underneath. Every structure was carefully labelled in Greek and Latin, Hebrew and Arabic in an attempt to standardize the naming of the body's anatomy.

◀ The murderer William Burke illustrated in this seventeenth-century engraving. His victims were supplied to Edinburgh Medical School so the students could dissect the bodies.

 ## GRAVE ROBBERS

When medical schools were set up in Europe during the seventeenth and eighteenth centuries, there was a growing shortage of bodies for anatomy lessons. So organized gangs of grave robbers removed bodies from new graves for students to cut up in classes.

It was only a short step from body snatching to murder. In Edinburgh, Scotland, an infamous series of anatomy murders occurred in 1827. These eventually led to the trial and execution of a labourer called William Burke (1792–1829). As fitting punishment, Burke's body was publicly dissected!

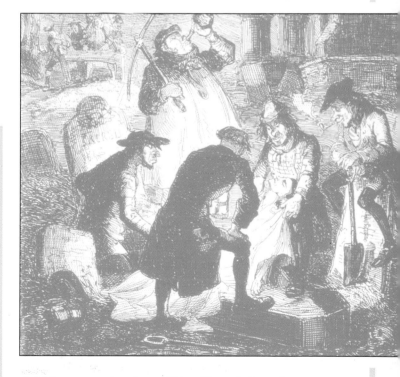

▲ This engraving from *The Chronicles of Crime* (London, Britain in 1887) shows body snatchers raiding a new grave to provide a fresh body for medical dissection.

⚙ CIRCULATION

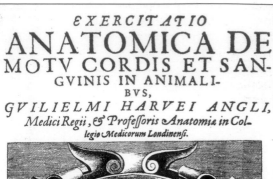

It is hard to imagine a time when doctors did not know how blood circulates around the body. But while explorers were sailing around the world on behalf of Elizabeth I of England (1533–1603), her physicians still did not know about circulation inside the human body. In 1628, William Harvey (1578–1657), physician to two British kings, published pioneering experiments on the circulation of blood. This was one of the first advances to take medicine out of the age of witchcraft and into the modern scientific era.

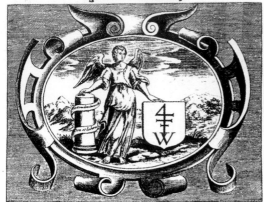

⚙ WILLIAM HARVEY AND THOSE WHO CAME AFTER

William Harvey was born in England on 1 April 1578. He went to school in Canterbury and to university at Cambridge. In 1598, he moved to the medical school in Padua, Italy, returning to England in 1604 to work at St Bartholomew's Hospital, London. Harvey began to give lectures about his experiments on circulation in 1616, but did not publish his results for another eleven years. His discovery was based on a series of experiments in humans showing that blood went around the body in a circle – flowing away from the heart through one set of blood vessels – the arteries – and back again through another set – the veins. Harvey showed that blood could only flow in one direction, and that a series of valves in the heart and blood vessels prevented it from moving back the way it had come.

Later in 1661, an Italian doctor, Marcello Malpighi (1628–1694), described the tiny blood vessels in the lungs, called capillaries. But it was Stephen Hales (1677–1761), a British clergyman and scientist, who developed the first instrument to measure the pressure of blood as it flowed through the arteries. In 1732, Hales described to the Royal Society in London how he had put a long glass tube into a horse's artery and attached it to a vertical brass pipe. The force of the animal's heartbeat pushed the blood to a height of 2.5 metres above the level of its heart.

► A patient recovers in intensive care following a heart operation. The patient is linked to a machine that helps with breathing. Various drips feed fluid and drugs directly into his blood stream. Other machines monitor the progress of his heart.

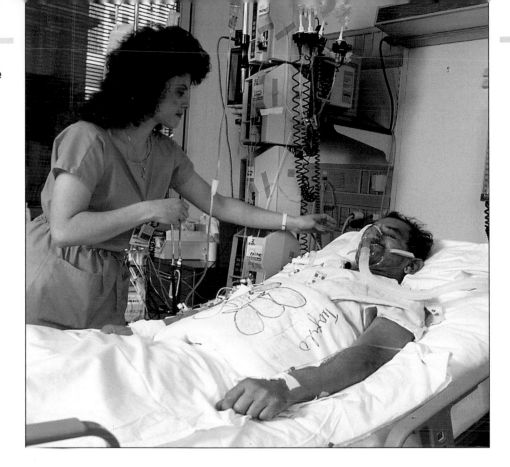

◄ The first page of William Harvey's book which was published in 1628 in Holland. In this book Harvey described the results of his experiments on human circulation.

▼ The heart pumps blood around the body in a never-ending cycle. The blood leaves the heart through the arteries and returns through the veins.

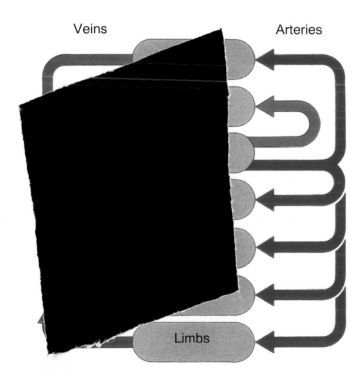

Veins   Arteries

Limbs

Red = plenty of oxygen
Blue = very little oxygen

Over the next 100 years, physicians began to describe diseases of the heart and circulation, and to try and treat them. In 1785, the British doctor and botanist William Withering (1741–1799), showed that the foxglove *Digitalis purpurea* was the vital ingredient of a herbal mixture used to treat a condition called dropsy – swelling in the limbs due to poor heart activity. *Digitalis* is used to this day in tablet form to make the heart work harder to pump blood around the body. Dozens of other heart and circulation drugs have been discovered since Withering did his research. Today, doctors can give people drugs to lower their blood pressure, to make their heart beat faster or slower, to help unblock their arteries and even to rescue their heart after a heart attack.

MICROSCOPES AND MICROBES

While great strides were being made to understand how the body worked, little progress was being made to stop the spread of disease. The main reason was that no one had much idea what caused plagues and epidemics. For centuries, infections were blamed on noxious gases, such as 'miasma' from rubbish dumps and cesspits, or vapours. The main obstacle to a more scientific understanding was that the killers responsible were invisible to the naked eye.

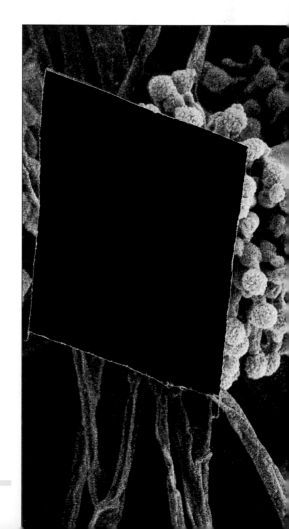

▼ The fungus *Aspergillus fumigatus*, which is found in dust, soil and vegetable material, is shown here as a false-colour picture produced by an electron microscope. The fungus causes allergic reactions and breathing problems.

The first microscopes were used in the middle of the fifteenth century. They were simple devices and are thought to have been developed by a number of people independently, including the Italian scientist, Galileo Galilei (1564–1642). A major step forward in medicine came in 1673, when the Dutch scientist Anthony van Leeuwenhoek (1632–1723) made a microscope that could magnify objects by up to 270 times their normal size. When he put saliva under the microscope, he could see rod and spiral-shaped microbes, which we now know are bacteria that live permanently in the mouth.

The arrival of the microscope almost immediately opened the eyes of doctors to bacteria, yeasts, fungi and other tiny organisms. Great progress was made between 1860 and 1900 in understanding infectious diseases. The French scientist, Louis Pasteur (1822–1895), showed that fermentation in wine, beer and milk was due to micro-organisms in the air, and not to something that appeared from nowhere, as it was previously thought. This work inspired the British surgeon, Joseph Lister (1827–1912), to use antiseptic methods during his operations. In March 1865, Lister operated for the first time using carbolic acid as an antiseptic. Wound infection, which was a daily hazard for nineteenth-century surgeons, failed to develop. However, it was some time before Lister's methods were widely accepted.

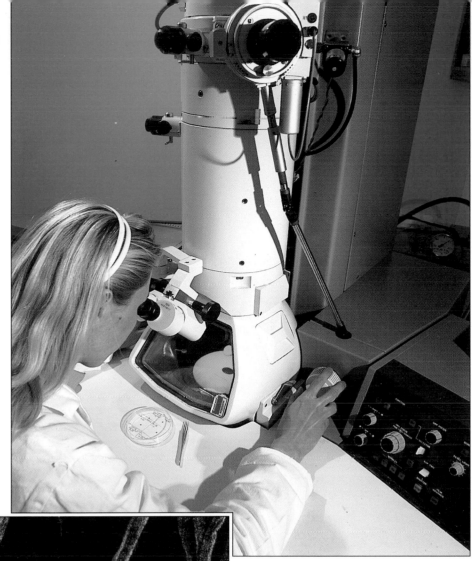

◄ A transmission electron microscope. This microscope can magnify objects up to several million times. A beam of electrons is fired down the tube of the microscope and passes through the specimen to a fluorescent screen. The image can be displayed on a television monitor or produced as a photograph. The beam is focused by electromagnets.

The world's first electron microscope was demonstrated in 1940 in Camden, New Jersey, USA. It was 10 feet high and weighed 700 pounds.

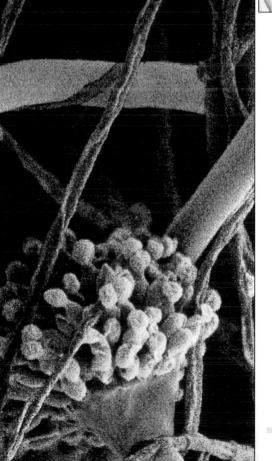

Scientists today can choose from a range of different types of microscope, depending on what they want to look at. A standard light microscope can be used to look at thin samples, usually stained with chemicals, mounted on glass slides. If a sample cannot be stained and is transparent (like most living cells) a special mirror can be added to give a dark background to the slide and make the sample show up brightly. Samples can be made to look extra bright by adding special dyes.

For the most detailed pictures, scientists now use electron microscopes. These use electrons instead of light to achieve far higher magnifications. The disadvantage is that this technique kills living tissue, so only dead samples can be examined. Since electrons are invisible to the naked eye, images have to be treated and photographed to get a picture.

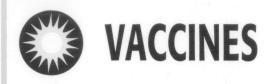

VACCINES

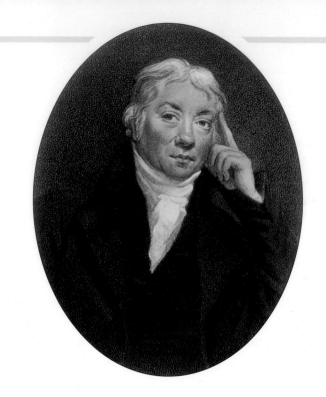

On 14 May 1796 a British doctor, Edward Jenner (1749–1823), took a small sample of infected tissue from the right hand of a dairy maid who had cowpox and injected it into the arm of an eight-year-old boy, called James Phipps. Over the next week, James developed small sores where he had been injected and felt a little unwell. But he soon got better. On 1 July 1796, Jenner injected James again – this time with a small amount of tissue from someone with smallpox. James remained healthy and lived to an old age.

▲ Edward Jenner, whose ideas on vaccination were at first ridiculed.

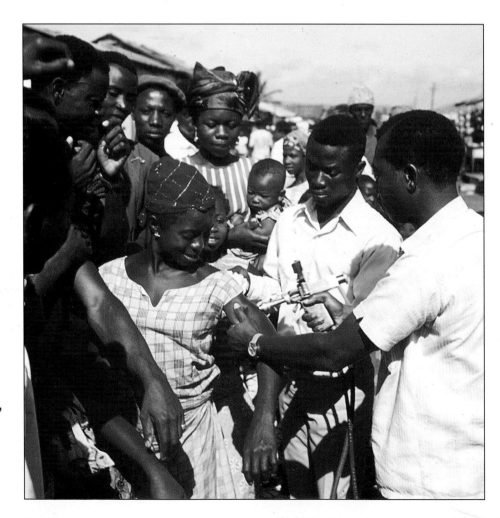

► In 1979, the World Health Organization declared that smallpox had been eradicated from the globe thanks to a massive vaccination programme, which reached the most remote parts of the Earth. Today, the virus is safely kept in only a handful of laboratories around the world.

Before Jenner's pioneering experiments, many people living in cities caught smallpox, and about one in five died from it. The disease is thought to have killed from about 200,000–600,000 people a year in Europe during the eighteenth century. It wiped out 3.5 million Aztecs after European armies infected with the disease invaded Mexico in 1519, and it killed about 6 million American Indians when settlers carried it to the North American plains in the late eighteenth century.

Jenner did not become an instant hero for his work – far from it. At first few people accepted his ideas. No one would publish his work and he had to pay to have his results printed. Previously, other doctors had injected people with small amounts of tissue from patients infected with smallpox, hoping this would protect them from later infection. Some people survived the injections, some died – exactly what happened in a real outbreak of smallpox. These doctors insisted that Jenner was wrong. One doctor who did try to confirm Jenner's work accidentally contaminated the cowpox vaccine with smallpox and got bad results. Over time, Jenner was proved right, and during the first half of the nineteenth century, people were vaccinated against smallpox in Italy, Turkey, the Middle East and beyond.

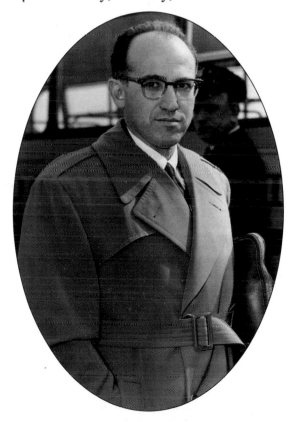

▲ Jonas Salk (1914–), an American scientist, who in 1954 developed the first vaccine against the virus disease, poliomyelitis. Poliomyelitis particularly affects children and young people but they can now be protected in infancy.

 MODERN VACCINES

A vaccine works by mobilizing the body's immune system to defend itself against attack by bacteria, viruses and other microbes. Today, vaccines are available against dozens of infections that used to be fatal, including poliomyelitis, tuberculosis, hepatitis and measles. A vaccine usually contains a small amount of the infectious organism, which has first been killed or specially treated to stop it from being dangerous. White cells in the blood attack the organism and learn how to identify it. Then, if they come into contact with it again during a real infection, they can quickly kill it. We still need new vaccines. For example, doctors are searching for a vaccine against the AIDS virus.

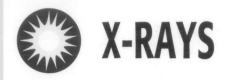

X-RAYS

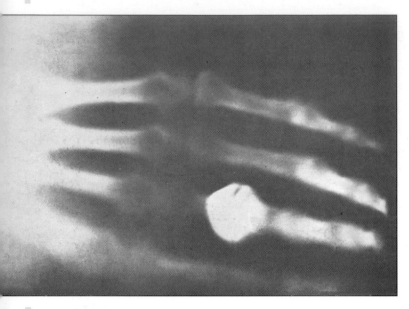

▲ The first ever X-ray of a human body was made by Wilhelm Röntgen of his wife's hand following his discovery of X-rays in 1895.

In November 1895 the German physicist, Wilhelm Röntgen (1845–1923), discovered how to see inside a body without having to open it up with a scalpel. He used X-rays to take pictures of the bones of his wife's hand. Unlike Edward Jenner, who had to wait years for his work to be accepted, news of Röntgen's discovery spread like wildfire. A few months after he reported his results at a meeting in Würzburg, Germany, scientists were taking X-ray pictures in other parts of Europe and in North America. Soon they had pictures not just of bones, but of intestines and other organs.

 CANCER TREATMENT

Modern cancer treatment uses high doses of X-rays to destroy tumours. This is called radiotherapy and it is often used to get rid of tumours that surgeons are unable to operate on, for example bone and brain tumours.

Narrow beams of X-rays are carefully aimed at the tumour from several directions at once. This means that the tumour gets a huge dose of harmful X-rays. But the healthy tissues that each beam passes through are exposed to a much smaller amount and are not affected.

▼ X-rays can be used to treat brain tumours. The rays focused on the tumour approach the head from many different directions. The tumour receives a high-level dose; the rest of the head receives only a low dose.

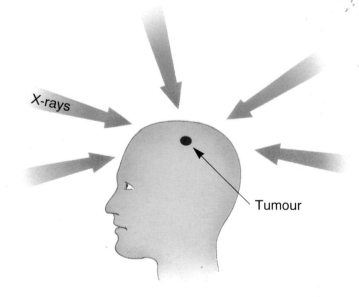

X-rays

Tumour

X-rays are high energy rays, invisible to the human eye, which can penetrate solid objects. When X-rays pass through the body, some tissues absorb them more than others. Dense tissues, such as bones, absorb a lot of rays whereas fatty tissues, which are watery, absorb few. What Röntgen discovered was that unabsorbed rays go straight through a body and will blacken a photographic plate if placed behind it. The plate stays white in places where X-rays haven't got through, because they have been absorbed by bones or other dense tissues on the way. The result is a picture in which solid parts of the body, such as bones, appear white and soft parts such as muscle look black.

Over 100 years ago X-rays were a huge advance. But they have turned out to be just the beginning. Researchers soon discovered they could get better pictures of the body's hollow tubes, such as the intestines, the airways and blood vessels, by injecting special dyes. These dyes absorb X-rays instead of letting them pass straight through. In 1973, scientists discovered a way of getting a computer to process dozens of X-rays at once to produce pictures of thin 'slices' of the human body – rather like a loaf of bread. This technique is called computerised axial tomographic, or CT scanning. CT scanners were originally introduced to get better pictures of the brain. But they are now widely used to detect tumours and other abnormal tissue in all parts of the body.

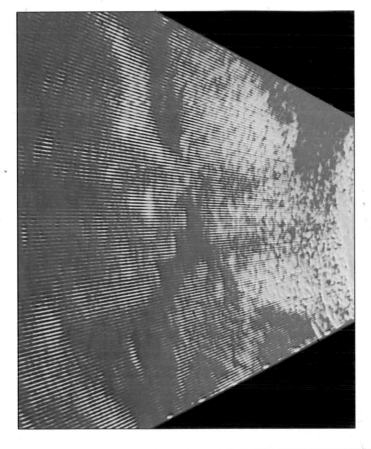

◀ An ultrasound picture of the face of an unborn baby after seven months of development. X-rays would be dangerous to use on an unborn child because they would interfere with its growth pattern.

X-rays have one important disadvantage: in high doses they can cause cancer. X-ray machines and CT scanners use tiny doses, but researchers have looked for ways of seeing inside the body without using X-rays at all. For example, doctors now use high-pitched sound waves to take pictures of babies in the womb before they are born. This is called ultrasound. Another technique, called magnetic resonance imaging (MRI), uses magnetic fields to produce vertical or horizontal pictures inside the body.

BLOOD GROUPS

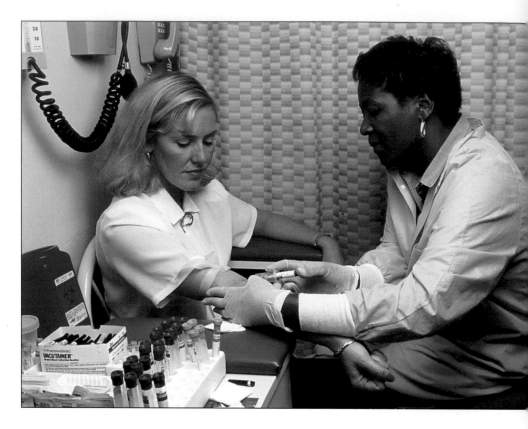

▶ Blood samples are commonly taken from a vein on the inside of the arm. First the blood flow is restricted by fastening a strap around the top of the arm. This makes the vein bigger. Then a hypodermic needle is inserted and blood drawn into a sterile syringe. Afterwards the sample is sent to a laboratory for testing. The doctor taking the blood sample wears latex gloves to prevent cross-infection.

Have you ever had a blood transfusion? Today, we take it for granted that if we lose a lot of blood in an accident or an operation, it can be replaced in hospital by a blood transfusion. But at the beginning of this century, people only had a blood transfusion as a last resort. It was very dangerous because doctors did not know before the transfusion whether the blood was suitable.

The first blood transfusion was given to a Parisian boy in the seventeenth century. In 1667 the French physician, Jean Baptiste Denys (1640–1704), transfused 340 grammes of lamb's blood into the boy. Remarkably, he survived. But a later patient of Denys – Antoine Mauroy – who was also given sheep's blood died. Madame Mauroy accused the doctor of murder. Denys was acquitted but the court said that no further transfusions could take place without official permission.

▶ A blood transfusion is the reverse of taking a blood sample. A tube is inserted into a vein in the arm, and the blood allowed to drip in from a bag supported above the patient's head.

The Austrian researcher Karl Landsteiner (1868–1943) finally paved the way for modern blood transfusion in 1901. He showed that human blood contains proteins, known as antibodies, which react to a second set of proteins, known as antigens, on the surface of red blood cells.

There seemed to be two types of antigen; some people's blood cells had one type of antigen, some another, some both, and some had none at all. The result was four different blood groups – A, B, AB and O. Mixing the groups together could be very dangerous. Give a patient blood of the right group, and a transfusion works every time. Give the person the wrong group and the result can be fatal.

 ## BLOOD GROUPS

Blood group	Can receive blood type	Antigens on red cells	Antibodies in plasma
O	O	none	A and B
A	A and O	A	B
B	B and O	B	A
AB	AB, A, B, O	AB	none

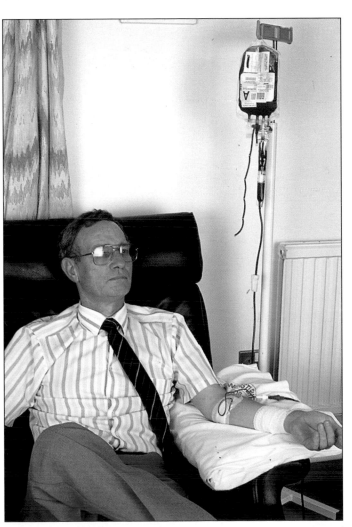

Since Landsteiner's work, other blood groups have been discovered. The most important of these is probably the rhesus group. In 1940, it was found that eight out of ten humans have an antigen on their red cells that rhesus monkeys also have – hence the name.

Most of the time it is unimportant whether you are rhesus positive or negative. However, if a rhesus negative woman has a rhesus positive baby, she may develop antibodies to the rhesus antigen during the pregnancy or at birth and this can be dangerous for that baby or later babies. Rhesus negative women are now given injections to destroy any harmful antibodies – usually after the birth and sometimes during the pregnancy.

INSULIN

The abnormally high sugar content in diabetic urine was first recorded in the seventeenth century by the British doctor Thomas Willis (1621–1675). But it was not until 1890 that researchers discovered that removing the pancreas from an animal gave it diabetes – a condition resulting in tremendous thirst, coma and eventual death.

Slowly, the cause of diabetes was discovered. In 1869, the German doctor, Paul Langerhans (1847–1888), described groups of cells in the pancreas, which became known as the Islets of Langerhans, and in 1901 an American doctor, Eugene Opie (1873–1971), realized that it was these cells that went wrong in diabetes.

Two groups of researchers – one in Bucharest, Romania, and the other in Toronto, Canada – raced to discover what was wrong with the Islet cells in people with diabetes. The Canadians won the race when in 1921, Frederick Banting (1891–1941) and Charles Best (1899–1978) discovered a hormone which they called insulin. It was the lack of this hormone that caused diabetes. Within a year people with diabetes were being treated and diabetic coma became a rare and unnecessary complication of the disease.

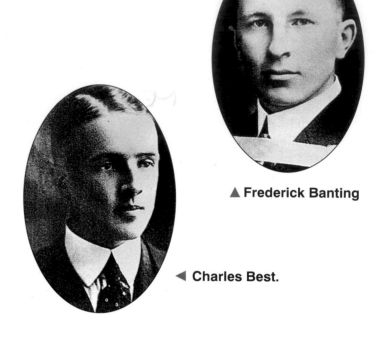

▲ Frederick Banting

◄ Charles Best.

▲ Charles Best was assigned to help Frederick Banting, who in 1922 was trying to discover a hormone from the pancreas. They succeeded not only in finding the hormone, but also in proving its link with diabetes. When Banting and the research director James McLeod (who had been on holiday) were awarded a Nobel Prize in 1923, Banting was furious and insisted on sharing his half with Best.

► The pancreas is a gland which is close to the stomach. It has two purposes. One is to produce digestive juices. The other is to produce the hormone insulin.

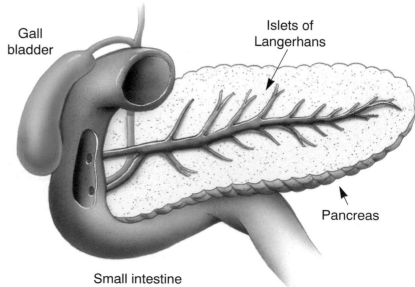

Gall bladder

Islets of Langerhans

Pancreas

Small intestine

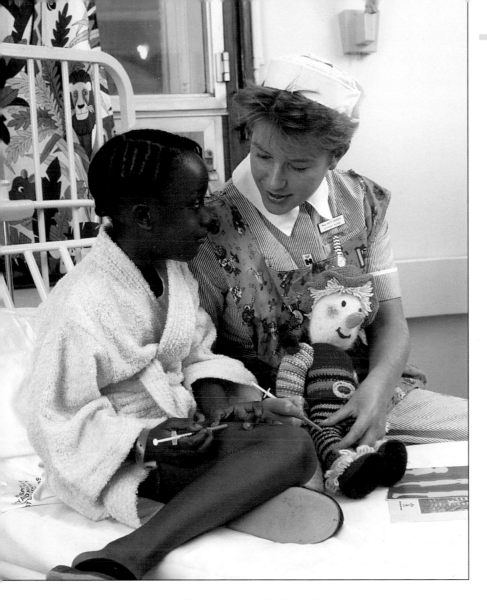

▲ Today young diabetics are taught how to inject themselves with insulin. Without insulin, sugar levels in the blood cannot be controlled.

✸ REPLACING HORMONES

Insulin is not the only hormone that can be replaced. People who do not have enough growth hormone, or thyroid hormone, can also have regular treatment.

When women reach the age of about fifty their bodies no longer produce the female sex hormones oestrogen and progesterone. This is called the menopause. Millions of women around the world now avoid hot flushes, depression and other miserable symptoms by using hormone replacement therapy (HRT). HRT also helps to protect women from developing brittle bones and heart attacks when they are old.

Insulin controls the amount of sugar in the blood. Too much sugar not only leads to coma and death, it also causes damage to the eyes, the kidneys and the nerves. Thanks to a lot of hard work over several decades, people with diabetes can today control their blood sugar levels so well that they can avoid these problems and lead virtually normal lives.

ANTIBIOTICS

The biggest chance discovery of the twentieth century is probably the discovery of penicillin in 1928. Alexander Fleming (1881–1955), a Scottish bacteriologist working at St Mary's Hospital, London, had been studying a type of bacterium that causes boils. He had carefully smoothed some of the bacteria on a small dish of nutrient jelly, and left it in his laboratory while he went away for his summer holiday.

During Fleming's absence, a fungus dropped on to the plate, and a cold spell of weather provided ideal growing conditions. The fungus released a substance later called penicillin, which prevented the bacteria on the dish from growing properly.

When Fleming returned from holiday, he found that bacteria growing near the fungus had dissolved. He was fascinated. Repeating his experiments, he found that penicillin was more effective against some types of bacteria than others, and he showed that it was not harmful to animals. But he did not realize just how important his discovery was. Fleming found penicillin a useful tool for his experiments, but never thought of using it to cure infections.

In 1939 the Australian pathologist, Howard Florey (1898–1968) and the British physicist and chemist Ernst Chain (1906–1979), working at Oxford University, turned their attention to penicillin. They purified a small amount and showed it could treat infections in animals.

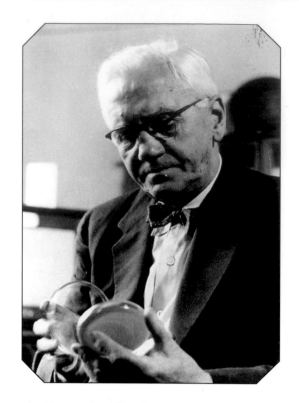

▲ Alexander Fleming examining dishes similar to those he used in 1928 when he discovered penicillin.

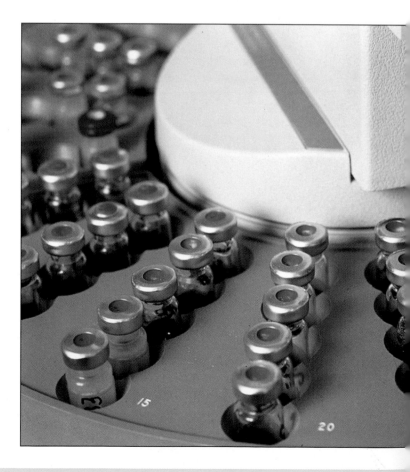

At last in 1941, thirteen years after Fleming's discovery, a small study began using penicillin on human beings. The penicillin was in short supply; it even had to be saved from patients' urine after it had passed through their bodies. But it worked. The Second World War was in progress and this made the research really urgent. American researchers helped to find a way to produce penicillin in the large quantities needed to treat injured servicemen with infected wounds. Other scientists worked out the chemical structure of penicillin, though it remained cheaper to produce the drug from fungi fermenting in huge vats than to make it in the laboratory.

In 1945, Fleming, Chain and Florey were jointly awarded a Nobel Prize for their penicillin research.

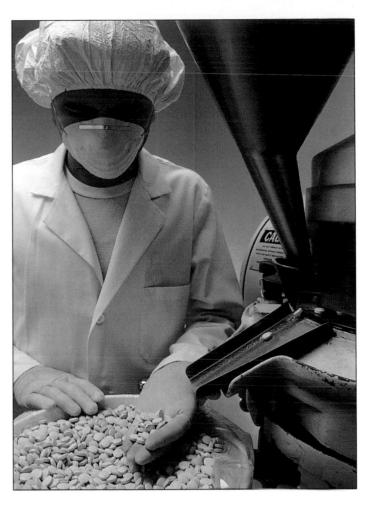

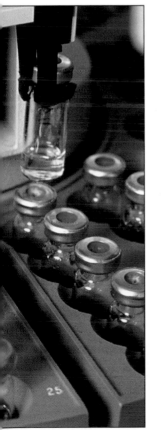

◀ These test samples are part of a research programme to find drugs that are active against antibiotic-resistant bacteria.

▲ Once a drug has been thoroughly tested, the production process is scaled up so the drug can be produced in large quantities for general sale.

AFTER PENICILLIN

The story of antibiotics did not end in 1945. Research is never as easy as that. Penicillin saved thousands of lives, but it was not long before some bacteria became resistant to its effects. In the fifty years since penicillin became a household name, many different types of penicillin have been produced.

Part of the problem arose because antibiotics were prescribed for minor infections when they were not really necessary. This gave the bacteria a chance to develop defence mechanisms against the drugs, making them ineffective when the infection was really serious. Today doctors are far more cautious and usually only prescribe antibiotics if they are really necessary.

Researchers are also working on the possibilities of finding drugs that stimulate the immune system to fight antibiotic-resistant bacteria.

TRANSPLANT IMMUNOLOGY

When the South African surgeon, Christiaan Barnard, performed the first heart transplant in 1967, he made history. The patient – a Cape Town dentist called Louis Washkansky – lived for just two weeks. Today, eight out of ten heart transplant patients can expect to live for at least five years. They owe their extra years to the skilled surgeons who perform their operations; and also to the men and women, whose names are not well-known, but who did the vital laboratory research in the 1940s and 1950s, making the first human transplant operations possible.

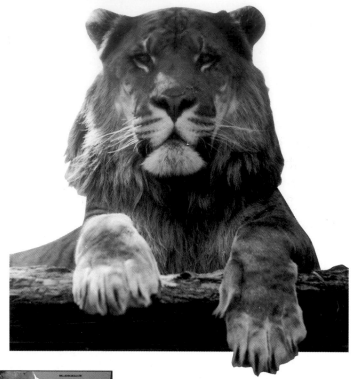

▲ This creature was born in a South African zoo, the result of crossing a South African lion with a Bengal tigress. Experiments in the cross-breeding of different species of animals are of interest to scientists studying immunology. In 1981 a sheep and a goat were successfully cross-bred in Japan.

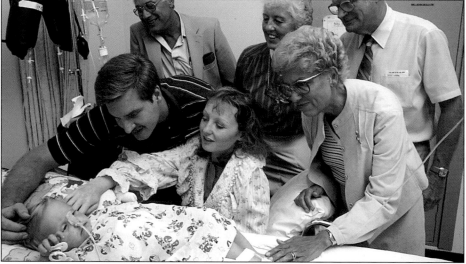

▲ Organ transplants between close relatives have a much higher chance of success. This child is recovering after an operation to transplant a kidney from his mother.

The first recorded attempts at organ transplants were made by the French surgeon, Alexis Carrell (1873–1955), during the early 1900s. He transplanted kidneys and hearts from one animal to another, but the organs did not work for long. The big problem for Carrell – and for all surgeons who have done transplants since – was a process which is now called 'rejection'. The defence cells in the blood of the person who receives the transplant 'realize' that the new organ is from someone else and they attack, and eventually destroy it.

During the 1940s and 1950s, four men – Peter Medawar (1915–1987) and Leslie Brent (1925–) from Britain, Rupert Billingham (1921–) from the USA, and Morten Simonsen from Denmark – carried out a series of vital experiments. They showed that if you put a piece of skin from one animal on to another, it will be rejected. Do it again, and it will be rejected more quickly. The animal's defence cells 'remember' what happened the first time. The next experiments put more pieces in the jigsaw. If skin was transplanted between twin animals, it wasn't rejected. Unrelated animals could also be made to accept transplants, if they were first given some defence cells from the donor animal.

Why were these experiments so important? They showed that it was possible to get around the problem of rejection, and encouraged other scientists to try and make anti-rejection drugs. Today, anyone who has a transplant is given a mixture of drugs to prevent their defence cells from rejecting the new organ. At first the person has to take big doses, but these can slowly be reduced as the years go by.

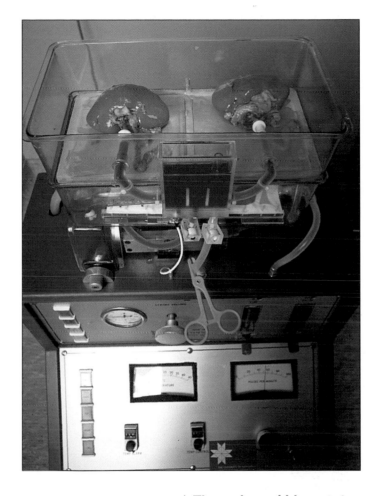

▲ These donor kidneys at the University of Minneapolis Hospital, USA, are being preserved before being transplanted into suitable patients.

 ## PIG ORGANS

There is a great shortage of human organs for transplantation, and doctors hope they may soon be able to use pig hearts, livers and kidneys instead. The work of Medawar and his colleagues has been very important here too. Today's researchers are building on the earlier work about rejection, to find ways to make humans tolerate organs from pigs.

They are breeding pigs with hearts which have some human antigens on them. Doctors hope that when these organs are transplanted into humans, the antigens will prevent them from being rejected.

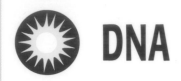

DNA

DNA stands for deoxyribonucleic acid. This molecule is present in the nucleus of every human cell and contains the instructions that pass on characteristics from one generation to the next. Its presence was first recognized in 1869, but no one knew what it did or what its structure was. Many people worked on DNA in the early part of the twentieth century, and by 1950 scientists knew that it was a complex molecule made up of simple building blocks. These are organized in a multitude of different ways to create the many different lifeforms that we have on Earth. What scientists needed to know was the structure of DNA and how it reproduced itself.

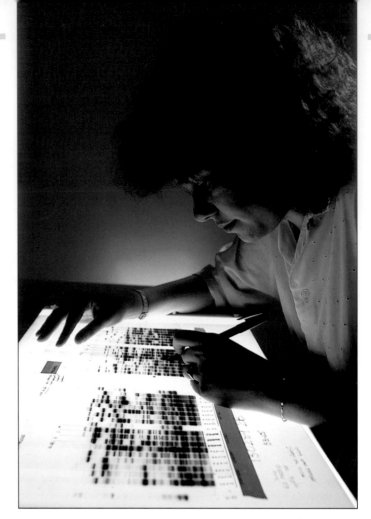

▲ DNA can be shown as a pattern of bands by a technique known as electrophoresis. These DNA 'fingerprints' are unique to each individual person but some bands are common to related people. DNA fingerprinting is used to prove conclusively that people are related, for example when immigrants to a country need to prove a family relationship.

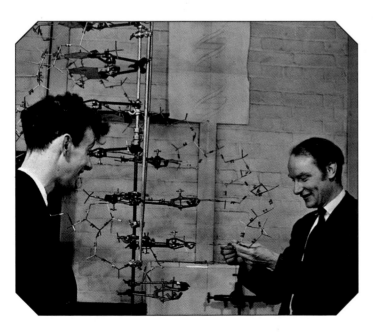

▲ James Watson (left) and Francis Crick in 1953 with their model for part of the DNA molecule.

In 1953, American biologist James Watson (1928–) and British scientist Francis Crick (1916–), both working at Cambridge University, England, made an intuitive breakthrough. Using X-ray data provided by British physicist Maurice Wilkins (1916–) and British crystallographer Rosalind Franklin (1921–1958), Watson and Crick worked out that the structure of the DNA molecule is like a rope ladder twisted into a spiral – a double helix. From this they were able to see how cells decode DNA to make the proteins which help decide a person's physical and mental make-up.

● WHAT NEXT?

In 1973 two American scientists, Stanley Cohen and Herbert Boyer, announced the results of the first successful piece of genetic engineering. They had managed to put together a piece of DNA made of genes from two different *Escherichia coli* bacteria. Soon, other scientists were mixing animal and microbe DNA. They found a way to make bacteria produce human insulin, and to make sheep produce human growth hormone.

Next came genetic fingerprinting – a revolutionary new technique discovered by British scientist Alec Jeffreys, during the mid-1980s. This technique enables detectives to identify suspects by matching the pattern of their genes to microscopic samples of body fluids left at the scene of a crime. The technique has also been used to settle paternity cases when people are not sure who is the father of a child. It is even being used to draw up family trees of the ancient Egyptian pharaohs, using cells from mummies that have been dead for 3,000 years.

The possibilities seem endless: new ways to diagnose and treat disease, and gene therapy to save people who are prone to cancer and heart disease may become reality within the next twenty to thirty years.

Once scientists knew the structure of DNA, they wanted to improve nature. Research into genetic engineering has led to a multi-billion dollar research industry. Stay-ripe tomatoes, frost-proof plants, genetic fingerprinting to catch criminals, gene therapy for children with cystic fibrosis are just a few of the scientific breakthroughs that would not have been possible without the knowledge of the structure of DNA.

▶ **This ram has a human gene incorporated in its DNA. This gene is responsible for the production of α-1-antitrypsin, a protein necessary to healthy people. It is passed on to the ram's offspring and the protein is produced in ewe's milk, from which it is extracted. The protein is used to treat hereditary deficiency in humans.**

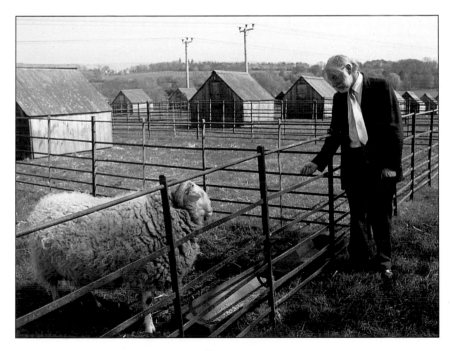

THE CONTRACEPTIVE PILL

Millions of women all over the world have control over their fertility – thanks to a small hormone pill which they take every day. Over the last thirty-five years it has become such an accepted part of modern living that it is called simply 'the pill'. Hormones are substances that help cells to function properly. The human female has two sex hormones: oestrogen ensures that eggs mature regularly in a woman's ovaries; and progesterone prepares the woman's womb each month to receive a fertilized egg. By controlling the levels of these hormones, we can control human fertility.

Before the start of the Second World War researchers had shown that injections of oestrogen and progesterone could prevent female rabbits from releasing eggs from their ovaries. The research was very slow because the hormones were in such short supply. An incredible four tonnes of pig ovaries were needed to get just twenty-five milligrammes of pure oestrogen.

▼ When using a contraceptive pill, a woman takes one pill a day for twenty-one days and then has seven pill-free days. Pills have the days of the week marked on their packaging. This shows whether or not the daily dose has been taken.

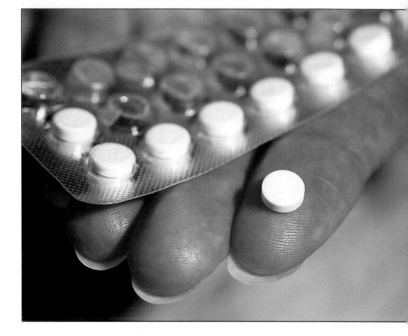

In 1939, Russell Marker, a chemist from Pennsylvania, USA, extracted progesterone from the roots of Mexican yams. Gradually, he improved the process and then joined forces with two European refugees to make hormones. They set up a company called Syntex, in Mexico. By the end of the war, Syntex was selling large amounts of hormones to other companies who manufactured medicines.

In 1949, a chemist called Karl Djerassi discovered how to make a progesterone-like chemical in the laboratory. This was taken further by the American biologist Gregory Pincus in 1956, when he tested the effect of progesterone on egg release in animals, and the Harvard gynaecologist, John Rock, who started testing it on women.

► After the Second World War, contraception became more widely available, enabling couples to control the size of their families. Most families today are smaller than the Canadian family shown here in 1962. There were eighteen children including seven sets of twins.

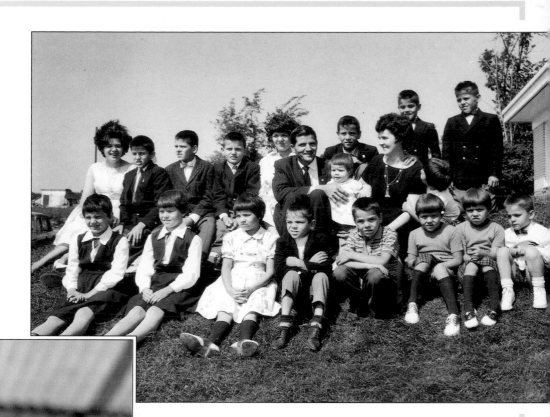

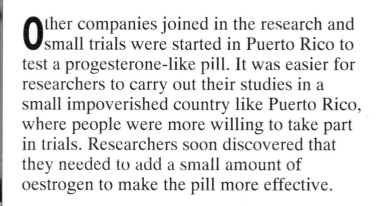

Other companies joined in the research and small trials were started in Puerto Rico to test a progesterone-like pill. It was easier for researchers to carry out their studies in a small impoverished country like Puerto Rico, where people were more willing to take part in trials. Researchers soon discovered that they needed to add a small amount of oestrogen to make the pill more effective.

Finally, the first contraceptive pill came on to the market in the USA in 1960, and in Britain a year later. Today, women can choose from many diffcrent types of pill. They all have smaller amounts of hormone than the first pills and fewer side effects.

◄ The population of China is more than a thousand million people. In efforts to reduce this, couples are restricted by law to have only one child, which makes reliable methods of contraception, such as the pill, a necessity.

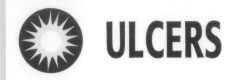 # ULCERS

If you get hydrochloric acid on your hands, it stings. The cells that line your stomach are much tougher than the skin on your hands, which is fortunate because they are exposed to hydrochloric acid most of the time. Hydrochloric acid helps to break down the food in your stomach. Some people, however, produce far too much hydrochloric acid, and it gradually eats away at their stomach cells forming an ulcer. An ulcer looks similar to a small fried egg, except it is white in the middle and red on the outside. Bad ulcers may bleed and this can be very dangerous.

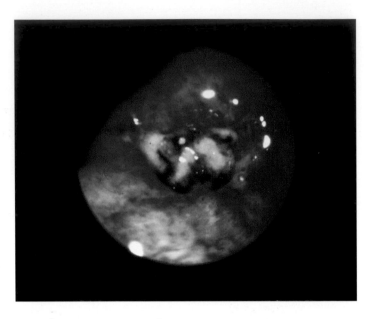

▲ Ulcers can be caused by an unsuitable diet, stress and certain drugs. This endoscope picture of a stomach ulcer shows bleeding in the crater at the centre of the ulcer.

▼ Some drugs are able to substitute themselves into active positions on cells so that they block their activity. The drug Tagamet is able to attach itself to acid-producing cells in the stomach, reducing the production of acid.

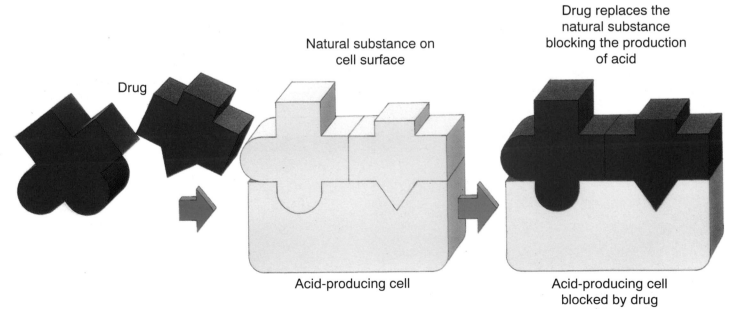

Drug

Natural substance on cell surface

Drug replaces the natural substance blocking the production of acid

Acid-producing cell

Acid-producing cell blocked by drug

Anyone who had an ulcer before 1976 took drugs to try and neutralize the excess acid in their stomach. If this did not work, they had an operation to cut the nerve that controls the acid production. It was a big operation and left them with no acid at all for digestion.

In 1976, the first of a new type of drug came on to the market. It could cure ulcers without surgery because it blocked an early stage of the process by which the stomach releases acid. The man behind the discovery was the drug specialist James Black (1924–). In the early 1970s, he became convinced that if he could design a drug that would bind to certain sites on the acid-producing cells, he could reduce the amount of acid they produced. Luckily for millions of people with ulcers, Black was right. The first of these so-called histamine-blocking (H2) drugs to come on to the market was named Tagamet. It made Black famous and the company he worked for very rich! Since 1976 several similar drugs have been produced, and hardly anyone has an operation for a stomach or intestinal ulcer any more.

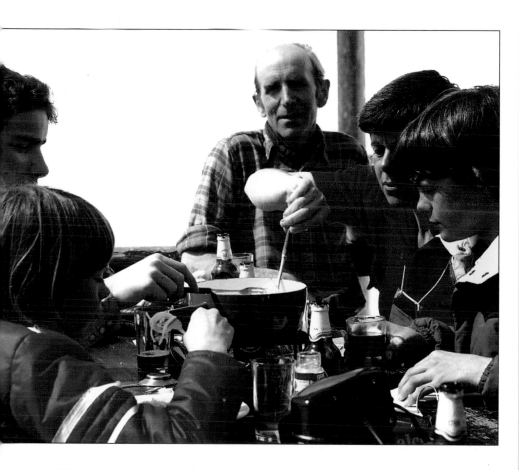

▲ Thanks to modern drugs, ulcer patients today can enjoy the same food as their friends and family.
In the past, sufferers ate a restricted diet and hoped that their ulcers would heal without surgery.

 A BUG IN THE WORKS

Most people thought Tagamet and its successors had closed the book on ulcer research. But they were wrong. In the last twenty years, doctors have found that although these drugs work very well, ulcers tend to come back when the drugs are stopped. In the last few years, scientists have made another discovery. They have realized that many people with ulcers have a bacterium in their stomach called *Helicobacter pylori*, and they have started to use antibiotics to get rid of it. The treatment works very well and now patients are often given H2 blockers to heal their ulcers, and antibiotics to prevent them from coming back.

MONOCLONAL ANTIBODIES

When your doctor takes a blood or urine sample from you and sends it to the laboratory, there's a good chance that it will be tested using monoclonal antibodies. Monoclonal antibodies are as useful to biologists as calculators are to maths students. No one could have realized how important they would be when, twenty years ago, two scientists, Cesar Milstein (1927–) and Georges Köhler (1946–1995), working at Cambridge University in Britain, stumbled across them almost by chance.

▶ **Cesar Milstein.**

▼ **Antibodies defend the body against invading infections.**

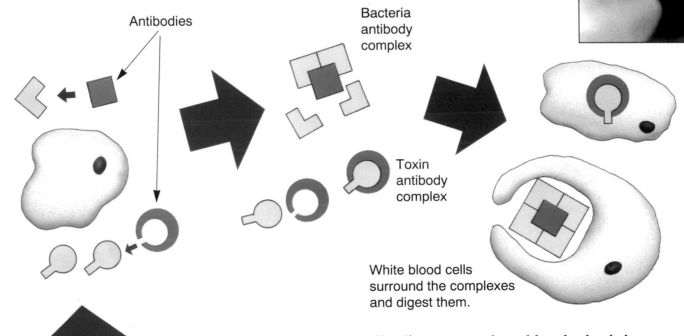

Antibodies

Bacteria antibody complex

Toxin antibody complex

White blood cells surround the complexes and digest them.

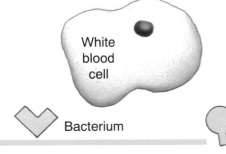

White blood cell

Bacterium

Toxins

Antibodies are produced by the body's immune system to attack anything in the body, including invading bacteria and viruses which they recognize as 'foreign'. Antibodies home in on proteins called antigens, which are like beacons on the surface of invading cells. Once the antibodies have made contact, they call in thousands of other cells to get rid of the invaders.

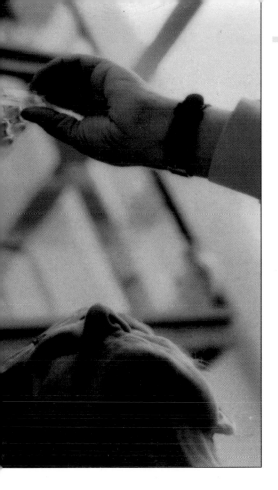

During the 1970s, researchers were keen to make use of the homing instincts of antibodies. They wanted to measure chemicals in fluid samples, to recognize diseased cells in the body and preferably even to carry drugs to them. Antibodies seemed a possibility. The problem was that cells only produce antibodies for short periods of time before they die, so they are difficult to obtain in any quantity.

Milstein and Köhler were doing research on the genes that make cells produce antibodies. Whilst mixing different types of cells they discovered that they had fused together antibody-producing cells with 'immortal' cancer cells. The resulting new cells could produce an endless number of copies, or clones, of the antibodies. These are now known as monoclonal antibodies or MABs. Today, researchers routinely create MABs to recognize all sorts of animal and human cells and chemicals. They are mainly used in laboratory tests to diagnose diseases. Some doctors use them to treat diseases. For example, anti-cancer drugs attached to monoclonal antibodies carry the drugs directly to cancerous tumours, avoiding normal, healthy cells.

▼ **A researcher separates monoclonal antibodies from cell culture, using a technique known as low pressure chromatography.**

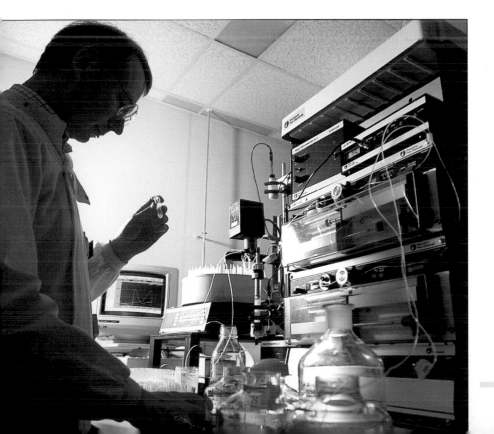

 LOST CHANCE

The discovery of monoclonal antibodies should have made millions of pounds for British science. But no one realized quite how important the discovery was. Normally, any important discovery is patented, which means it is put on an official register alongside the name of the person who did the work. Anyone who wants to use the process later on has to pay the discoverer.

No one patented MABs, so anyone can use them free of charge. In 1984, Milstein and Köhler won a Nobel Prize for their work.

TEST-TUBE BABIES

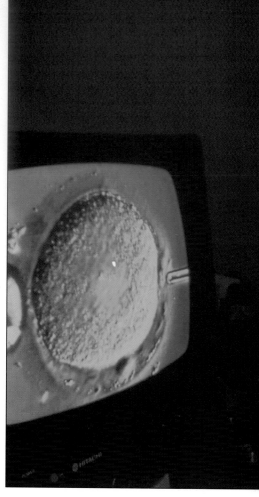

Louise Brown, born in 1978, was the world's first test-tube baby. She was the result of years of research by two doctors, Patrick Steptoe (1913–1988) and Robert Edwards (1925–), who worked at Cambridge University in England. Since then thousands of couples, who previously could not have children, have left hospital with healthy babies. The technique, which Steptoe and Edwards pioneered, is called in-vitro fertilization (IVF) and it can be used to help both women who cannot conceive and men who cannot produce enough sperm to fertilize their partner's eggs.

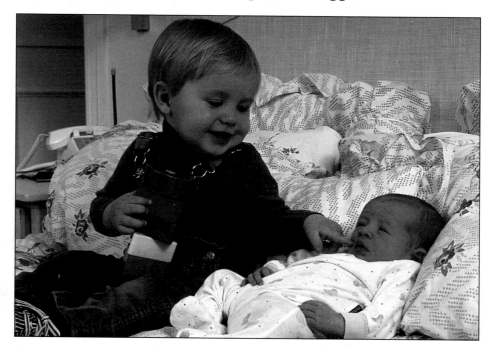

◀ These twin boys David (left) and Nicholas (right) were conceived on the same day by IVF, but were born a year and a half apart. Half the batch of fertilized eggs were implanted in their mother's womb producing David in 1987. The remainder were frozen and then used for a second implant producing Nicholas in 1989.

The first stage of IVF involves giving the woman special drugs to make her ovaries produce as many eggs as possible. These are then removed in hospital during a small operation, and mixed with sperm from the woman's partner. They are kept very carefully in just the right fluid mixture so that a sperm fertilizes each egg. To encourage a successful pregnancy, several of these fertilized eggs are then put back into the Fallopian tubes or the womb of the woman and left to grow normally. Any spare embryos are carefully frozen and stored so they can be used at a later date.

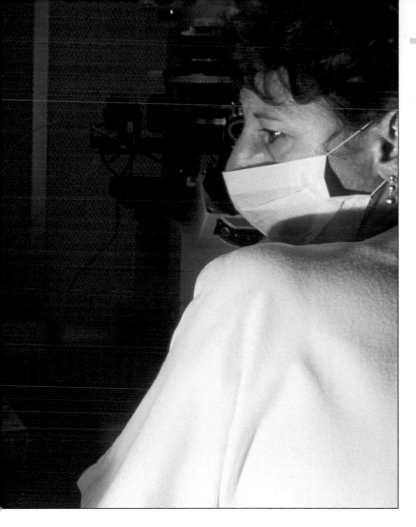

Working with a monitor attached to a microscope, a researcher controls the injection of a sperm cell into an egg. A pipette is used to hold the egg steady; a needle is inserted to inject the sperm cell. The technique ensures fertilization without wasting millions of sperm.

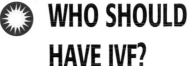

WHO SHOULD HAVE IVF?

The ability to 'make babies' in the laboratory has brought ethical problems. Some couples in their fifties and sixties have wanted a child and the woman has been treated with IVF. But so late in life, bodies are less fit, and there is a good chance that the parents will die while their children are still young.

Another problem has arisen because the fertilized eggs do not have to be put back into the woman who produced the eggs. When miscarriage is a problem some couples have chosen to pay another woman to give birth to their baby. After the birth, carriers have sometimes refused to give up the child.

There are now many variations on the original IVF technique. For example, some couples choose gamete intra-fallopian transfer (GIFT); this is simpler than IVF. The eggs are removed from the ovaries, and put into the womb straight away with some sperm. Fertilization then occurs inside the woman, not in the laboratory.

IVF can also help when the man does not produce enough sperm. To ensure fertilization inside a woman's body, it is necessary for a man to produce millions of sperm to make sure that at least one is successful in fighting its way up through the womb to the egg. In a laboratory test-tube it is much easier, so only a few sperm are needed.

THE CYSTIC FIBROSIS GENE

Cystic fibrosis is the most common, serious, inherited disease that we know. People who have the condition make thick mucus in their lungs and this clogs their airways, making it hard to breathe. They also have problems digesting and absorbing food because of mucus in their gut. On average, one in every twenty-five people have a copy of the faulty gene which leads to cystic fibrosis. They do not have any breathing or digestive problems and are completely well. But if they have a child with someone who also has a copy of the faulty gene, the baby can inherit both copies and will be born with cystic fibrosis.

For years researchers tried to find the faulty gene. They knew it was somewhere amongst the 100,000 genes on the twenty-three pairs of human chromosomes. But where? At first it was like looking for a word in the dictionary but not knowing how to spell it.

▶ Children with cystic fibrosis have regular physiotherapy at home, backed up by visits to hospital clinics. Parents are shown simple exercises that will help minimize the effects.

▼ A doctor and a genetic counsellor explain to potential parents the risks of passing on genetic ailments.

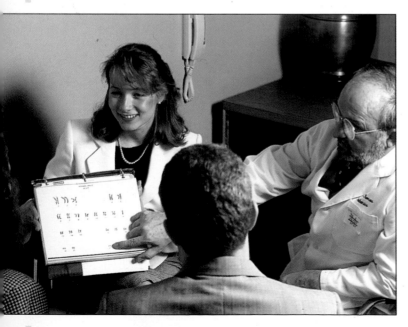

Three key groups of researchers – in Canada, the USA and Britain – were at the forefront of the research. By 1984, 20 per cent of the several million sequences of DNA on human chromosomes had been checked for the cystic fibrosis gene and ruled out. By 1985, 40 per cent had been checked and cleared. New groups of researchers, all in the USA, joined the race. But it was a Danish group, led by Hans Eiberg, who made the first breakthrough when they worked out that the cystic fibrosis gene was situated close to the gene for an enzyme called paraoxonase. The problem was that no one was sure whether the paraoxonase gene was on chromosome seven, eight or eighteen.

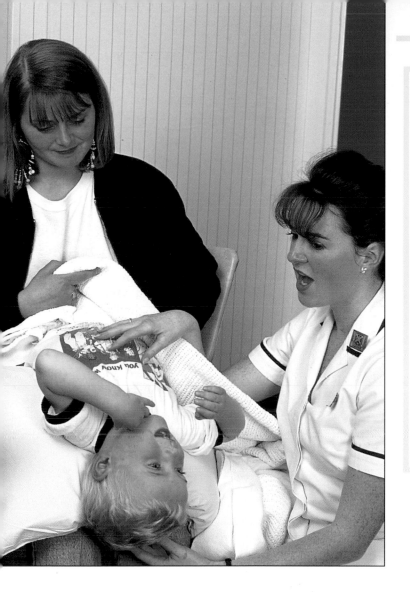

WHO WANTS TO KNOW?

The cystic fibrosis gene was the first of several recent discoveries. Scientists now know the whereabouts of the gene for muscular dystrophy – the inherited, muscle-wasting disease – and the gene for the inherited brain disease, called Huntington's chorea.

But such discoveries are not always welcome. Some people do not want to know if they have inherited a gene which could kill them, especially if there is no cure for their disease. They do not want a death sentence hanging over them or their children.

Some scientists are very worried about where this sort of research will lead. They are afraid that people with faulty genes will be penalized when it comes to getting jobs, buying a house or taking out life Insurance.

▼ **The cystic fibrosis gene is located about half-way along chromosome 7.**

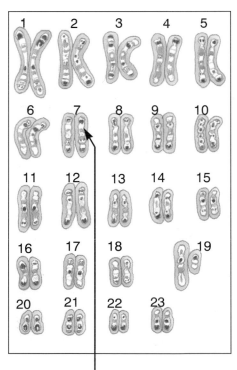

Cystic fibrosis gene

In November 1985, six important research papers were published all pointing to the same position for the cystic fibrosis gene – the middle of the long arm of chromosome seven. The research now became a competition. In the early days, the groups had co-operated and shared data, but in the final stages of the race, they were reluctant to exchange information. Finally, in August 1989, Francis Collins in Michigan, USA, and Lap-Chee Tsui and Emmanuel Buchwald in Toronto, Canada, announced that they had pinpointed the cystic fibrosis gene. The news flashed around the world. The discovery was extremely important. It meant that researchers could design a test to find carriers of the faulty gene. It could also be used to test unborn babies in the womb to see if they would have the disease.

In 1993, the first attempts at gene therapy for cystic fibrosis were made by researchers in the USA but it could be a number of years before they discover the best technique.

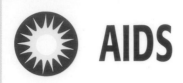# AIDS

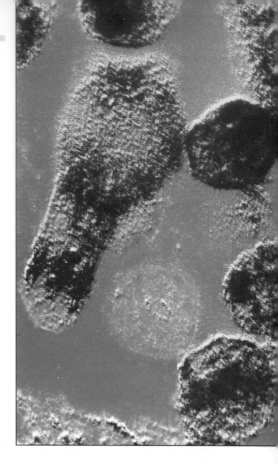

When the first reports of AIDS surfaced in June 1981, the disease did not even have a name. Two Los Angeles doctors had noticed a mysterious outbreak of an unusual lung infection in a group of young gay men. Next came reports of a very rare form of skin cancer – again in young homosexual men. Gradually, the pieces fell into place. Something was destroying their immune systems, making them prone to several rare, often fatal infections, and to the skin cancer called Kaposi's sarcoma. The disease was given a name – acquired immune deficiency syndrome (AIDS). But what was the cause?

Early in 1982, the American virologist, Robert Gallo (1937–), suggested that AIDS might be caused by a type of virus called a retrovirus. Gallo and his team had already discovered two retroviruses that cause rare types of human leukemia. They suggested that perhaps a similar sort of virus could cause AIDS.

▲ This false-colour picture, taken with an electron microscope, shows particles of the AIDS virus inside a white blood cell. Once inside the cell, the viral genetic material (the red colour inside the orange spheres) converts to DNA and takes over the DNA of the host cell.

▶ The stricken white blood cell begins to make copies of the AIDS virus, which then burst out of the cell wall, eventually destroying their host.

 ## RETROVIRUSES

These are unusual viruses in that they are made of the genetic material, ribonucleic acid (RNA), instead of DNA. In most viruses, and indeed in human cells, RNA is the messenger taking instructions from the DNA for making proteins. In retroviruses, the virus RNA is first converted into DNA before messenger RNA can start protein manufacture.

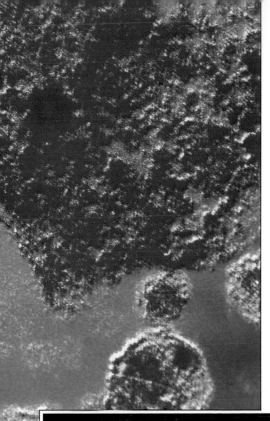

In Paris, a group of virologists, led by Luc Montagnier (1932–), were also interested in retroviruses. In 1983, they were sent a sample of cells from a patient in the early stages of AIDS. For days they tested the sample and eventually they saw tell-tale signs that RNA was being converted into DNA. This suggested that there was a retrovirus in the sample, and that this retrovirus was killing the white blood cells which it had infected. A month after they had been sent the original sample, they had a few fuzzy photographs of the virus.

Samples of virus went back and forth between Gallo and Montagnier. The French virologists were convinced they had found an entirely new virus. Gallo's group was sure it was related to the viruses they had already linked to leukemia. Eventually the Americans decided that it was the AIDS virus.

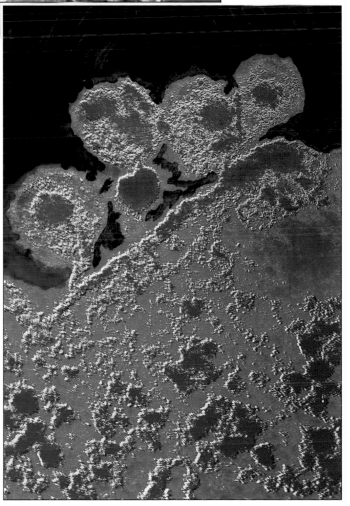

It was the start of a long and bitter battle between the French and American researchers over who discovered the AIDS virus, and who should own the patent for the AIDS tests that were later developed. The problem was solved by an agreement in March 1987, which was announced jointly by Ronald Reagan, president of the USA, and Jacques Chirac, prime minister of France. Gallo and Montagnier were to share the credit for the discoveries, and most of the royalty money to come from the research was to go into an AIDS research foundation.

☀ NEW FRONTIERS

Cancer, heart disease, dementia and arthritis are just some of the twentieth-century diseases that are still incurable. Much more is known about them now, at the end of the century, than was known at the beginning, but we are still waiting for the vital breakthroughs which could bring those elusive cures.

In industrialized countries, cancer has replaced infection as the leading cause of death. Research has already shown us some of the causes. For example, smoking may lead to lung cancer, too much sun may result in skin cancer, and a rich, fatty diet, low in fruit and vegetables, seems to be linked to bowel and breast cancers.

Doctors know that some people are more likely to get cancer than others. These people have faulty genes which can change normal healthy cells into malignant ones. Now scientists are trying to discover how this process happens. Only then will they be able to switch off the cancer genes and start to reduce the number of people who die from this terrible disease.

▶ **A researcher studies the genetic process of ageing for** *Project Chronos,* **at the Centre for the Study of Human Polymorphism in Paris, France. This project involves mapping the genes of people who have reached extreme old age (over 100 years), to understand the genetic process of ageing. The research may provide therapies to prolong life.**

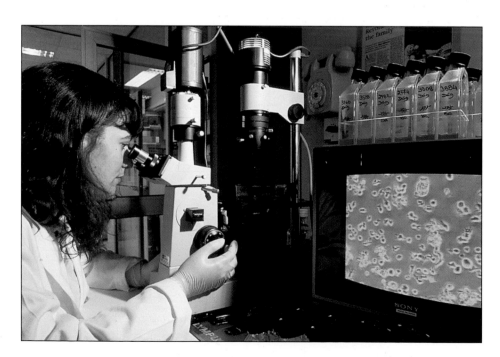

There is no point in living longer if you spend the later years confused and frightened, or in pain. Alzheimer's disease and other forms of dementia have become health problems because people live longer today. Researchers are slowly finding out why the nerves in the brain become tangled and diseased in some people, making them unable to think clearly when they grow older.

Most people who live into their seventies and eighties cannot move about as easily as they get older. Their joints become stiff and painful because the lining inside the joints wears out. This disease is called arthritis. Sufferers can only take painkillers and do their best to keep mobile, while researchers continue to search for a way to block the cells that damage the joints.

▶ AIDS researchers wear full protective clothing, consisting of cap, gloves, gown and mask, when working on samples infected with the AIDS virus. Laboratories used for highly dangerous biological research are protected by steel air-locks and decontamination rooms with twenty-four hour security and contamination alarms. These necessary safeguards add to the cost of the research.

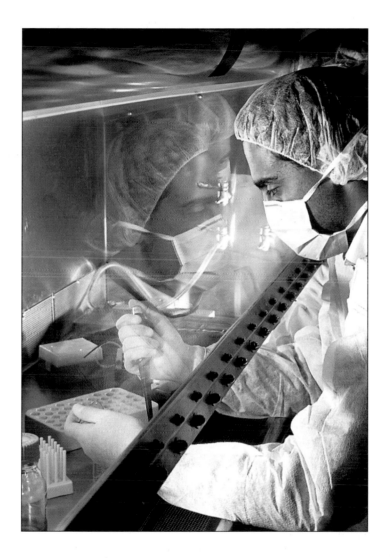

Millions of pounds are going into the research for a cure for AIDS – a disease that is killing more people in Africa and Asia than anywhere else in the world. But any drugs or vaccines, which may result from this research, may be too expensive for the people who need them most. Discoveries in medicine are always exciting. But the biggest thrill will come when patients all around the world feel the benefit.

TIMELINE OF ADVANCE

Here are some of the people, discoveries, inventions and improvements that have brought the standards of health care we have today.

Ancient Egyptians Egyptian embalmers in about 2000 BC were familiar with the internal organs of the human body because they removed all but the heart before mummifying corpses. They also practised trepanning (removing a portion of skull bone) to relieve pressure on the brain caused by damaged skulls.

Ancient Greeks Hippocrates and his followers around 400 BC started a more ordered approach to medicine by examining their patients and watching how they responded to treatment. They also laid down a code of ethics by which they would practise, promising not to harm their patients deliberately.

Medieval Europeans Between 1100 and 1300, progress in medicine was inhibited by the power of the Church. Doctors were not allowed to use dead humans for research and had to make do with animals. Much of what happened to people was believed to be 'God's will' and could not be changed.

Andreas Vesalius A Belgian anatomist (1514–1564) who greatly advanced the science of anatomy by publishing a book containing excellent descriptions of the bones and the nervous system. These were illustrated by magnificent drawings of muscle dissections by Jan Stephen van Calcar. Vesalius made sure that the names of different parts of the body were translated accurately into the commonly used languages of the time.

William Harvey An English doctor (1578–1657) who worked out that blood was pumped out of the heart by way of the arteries, passed through the flesh and returned to the heart through the veins. His ideas opened the way for new treatments for heart and circulatory problems. Before his time people believed that blood flowed from the heart and was absorbed by the body as food.

▼ **William Harvey**

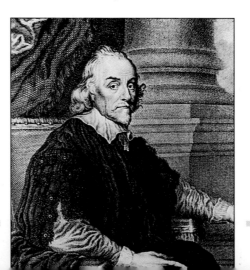

Anthony van Leeuwenhoek A Dutch scientist (1632–1723) who worked as a clerk in a cloth warehouse until 1654. He devised the first powerful optical microscope and made a series of pioneering discoveries relating to blood corpuscles, sperm and the circulation of the blood. Once doctors could see infection-causing microbes, they could begin to find ways of combating them.

Edward Jenner The British doctor (1749–1823) who performed the first attempts at vaccination, using material from people infected with cowpox to immunize others against the much more serious infection of smallpox.

Louis Pasteur An important French scientist (1822–1895) who is regarded as the founder of microbiology. He showed that infections were caused by organisms in the air and did not spontaneously appear from nowhere. With outstanding success he tackled silkworm disease, growths in beer, splenic fever and fowl cholera. He developed vaccines against anthrax and rabies. In 1888, the Institut Pasteur was founded in Paris for treatment of rabies. Today, it is an important centre for medical research.

Joseph Lister An English surgeon (1827–1912) who revolutionized the effectiveness of surgery in 1865 by introducing procedures for the use of antiseptics. Before this time, patients were quite likely to die because of infections that entered open wounds during and after surgery.

Wilhelm Röntgen The German physicist (1845–1923) who discovered X-rays. His breakthrough meant that fewer people needed operations to find out what was wrong with them, and led to further twentieth-century discoveries of ways to take accurate pictures of organs deep inside the body.

Karl Landsteiner An Austrian researcher (1868–1943) who discovered blood groups, paving the way for blood transfusion. Until he showed that there are four broad groups of blood – O, A, B, and AB – it was not possible to safely replace lost blood, and many people bled to death after accidents or operations.

Frederick Banting A Canadian doctor (1891–1941) who with **Charles Best** (1899–1978) discovered in 1921 that the hormone insulin, made in the pancreas, is responsible for the amount of sugar in the blood-stream. Today, millions of people with diabetes all over the world rely on injections of insulin to keep their blood sugar levels under control.

▼ Louis Washkansky is seen here in intensive care after Christiaan Barnard had successfully operated to give him a new heart in 1967.

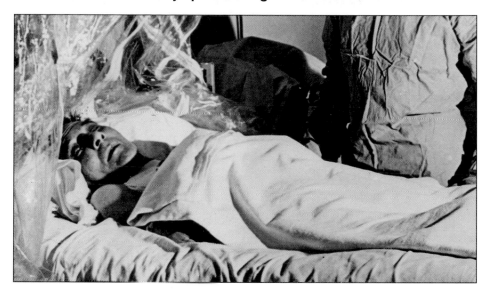

Alexander Fleming A British bacteriologist (1881–1955) who, in 1928, made the chance discovery of penicillin – an antibiotic which is used to this day to treat bacterial infections.

Howard Florey An Australian pathologist (1898–1968) who, working with the British biochemist **Ernst Chain** (1906–1979), discovered and purified penicillin, developed ways of making it on a large scale, and conducted the first clinical trials.

James Watson The American biologist (1928–) who, with the British scientist **Francis Crick** (1916–), discovered the structure of DNA. The discovery took place in 1953 while Watson and Crick were working at Cambridge University, England. Their work opened the way for genetic engineering and gene therapy during the 1970s, 1980s and 1990s.

Jonas Salk An American scientist (1914) who developed a vaccine for poliomyelitis in 1954. Until this time there was no effective defence against the disease. In 1950 a severe polio epidemic had swept across America, and in 1952 Belgium, Germany and Denmark also suffered epidemics. The Salk vaccine quickly became a routine treatment for young children preventing further epidemics in Europe and North America.

Christiaan Barnard A South African surgeon (1922–) who carried out the first successful heart transplant operation on 3 December 1967 at the Groote Schuur Hospital in Cape Town. The patient, **Louis Washkansky,** later died of pneumonia after his resistance to infection had been lowered by drugs administered to prevent him rejecting the new heart. Today many organs of the body can be safely transplanted.

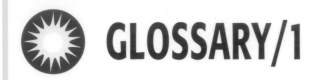 **GLOSSARY/1**

A ready-reference guide to many of the terms used in this book.

Antibiotic A drug that can kill bacteria.

Antibody A chemical produced by the body to fight infection and other invading substances.

Antigen A substance (usually a protein) which is recognized and attacked by an antibody.

Antiseptic A substance which reduces the growth of (but may not destroy) bacteria and other microbes.

Artery A blood vessel which carries blood away from the heart.

Bacterium (plural bacteria) A type of single-celled micro-organism, larger than a virus, which can live in animals or plants, or on its own. Some bacteria cause diseases.

Bile A dark yellow substance made in the liver which is important for digesting fat.

▶ **Although cells have different functions, most animal cells contain the common features shown in this typical cell, such as the nucleus, the membrane, mitochondria and organelles.**

Cancer This is a disorder of the process of growth, development and repair of cells, which causes the production of mutant cells. New tissue grows in a purposeless and uncontrolled way. Cancer cells spread to distant parts of the body.

Capillary The smallest blood vessel found in the circulatory system.

Cell The smallest living part of any living thing, cells can repair and reproduce themselves. Animals have millions of cells which do many different jobs. Cells can be grown and kept alive in the laboratory for long periods.

Chromosome A structure found in the nucleus of animal and plant cells. It is made up of DNA (which carries the genes) and protein. Humans have twenty-three pairs of chromosomes. These are usually only visible as separate structures when the cell is dividing, because normally they are curled up to prevent damage.

Clone A copy of a plant or organism that has been produced asexually.

Cowpox A virus infection in cattle which is related to smallpox and may cause mild symptoms in humans.

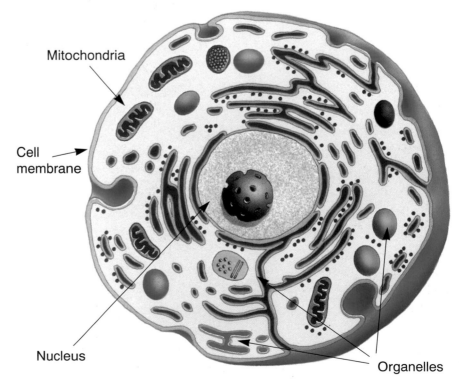

Mitochondria

Cell membrane

Nucleus

Organelles

Diabetes A disorder in which a person cannot control the amount of sugar in their bloodstream because the hormone, insulin, is not produced in the right quantities by the pancreas. Diabetes is one of the earliest recorded diseases being mentioned in an Egyptian papyrus dated around 1500 BC.

DNA (deoxyribonucleic acid) A substance in nearly all living things that contains the instructions for growth. DNA has the form of a double helix with the genes arranged in a linear pattern. DNA is found in the chromosomes in the nucleus of a cell.

Drug A substance which changes some aspect of the way the body functions. When used for medical purposes, drugs treat diseases and disorders bringing relief to the sufferer. Drugs misused for their pleasurable side-effects can cause serious harm and death.

Electrons The tiny negatively charged parts of an atom which act as carriers of electricity. Electrons are responsible for many phenomena such as lightning, electricity, radio waves and X-rays. The forces and energies of electrons are used in many kinds of laboratory equipment.

Embryo This is the name given to a human offspring between two and eight weeks after conception.

Ethics A moral code or set of rules for living.

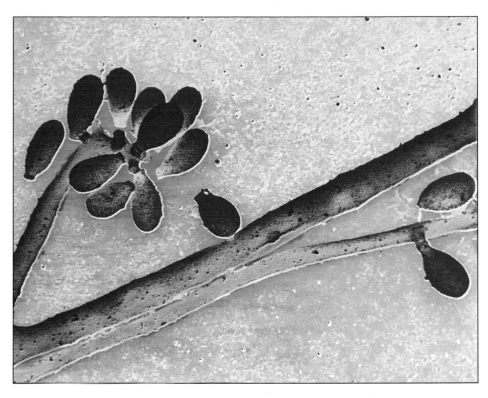

▲ This electron micrograph shows the fungus *Sporothrix schenckii* which grows in moss and bark. Florists and gardeners are vulnerable to infection by the fungus through open wounds on their hands. The infection can spread to the lungs and joints.

Fungus A member of a large group of living organisms like plants but without roots, stems or chlorophyll. Many are one-celled, microscopic, but larger than bacteria and these, or spores of the larger fungi, can cause disease.

Gene A section of DNA that carries the instructions for making an enzyme or other protein. All the genes of an organism are known as the genome.

Fallopian tubes Tubes that connect the ovaries to the womb, and along which the eggs travel.

Gynaecologist A doctor who treats diseases affecting the female sex organs.

Helix A spiral structure like a corkscrew.

Hepatitis A virus infection of the liver, the organ which changes digested food into products useful to the body.

Hormones Substances in plants and animals that help their cells function properly. Examples are insulin and oestrogen.

Immune system The organs, cells and molecules that recognize and get rid of harmful and 'foreign' substances that invade the body.

Leukemia A cancer of the white blood cells causing uncontrolled reproduction of the cells.

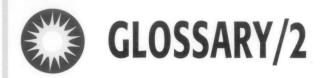
Measles A disease caused by a virus. It can be serious in young children because it allows bacteria to infect the lungs and ears. Today a vaccine is available that is given to children in early infancy.

Microbe Any type of micro-organism, including bacteria and viruses.

Micro-organism Any organism that is invisible to the human eye.

Miscarry To give birth before a baby is developed enough to survive.

Oestrogen The female hormone that makes eggs mature and stimulates secondary sexual characteristics such as breasts and pubic hair.

Ovary This is the female reproductive organ where eggs are made. Female human beings have two ovaries which release fertile eggs on alternate months.

Phlegm According to ancient myth, this is one of the four substances that controlled disease in the body. In modern terms, it is mucus-containing saliva.

Poliomyelitis (polio) A disease caused by a virus that attacks the nerves in the spinal chord. It affects mostly children and young adults and results in paralysis. Today children can be protected by regular doses of oral vaccine.

Progesterone The female sex hormone that prepares the womb each month to receive a fertilized egg.

RNA (ribonucleic acid) The substance that helps translate DNA into proteins. In some viruses, RNA is the genetic material itself.

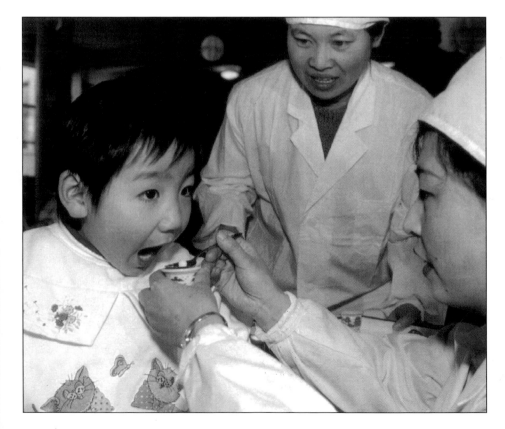

◄ **Chinese health workers administer the anti-polio vaccine in January 1995. This is part of a massive two-stage immunization programme aimed at 100 million Chinese children.**

Smallpox A usually fatal viral disease, eradicated from the Earth in 1979 by a worldwide vaccination programme. It involved a fever and blisters which left permanent scars on those who survived infection.

Tuberculosis An infectious wasting disease which occurs throughout the world. It is caused by bacteria and can affect the lungs, the bones, the joints and the central nervous system. It flourishes wherever undernourished people are crowded together in poor living conditions with inadequate health care.

Tumour An abnormal lump of cells growing on or in a body.

Thyroid A gland in the neck that controls the speed at which cells work.

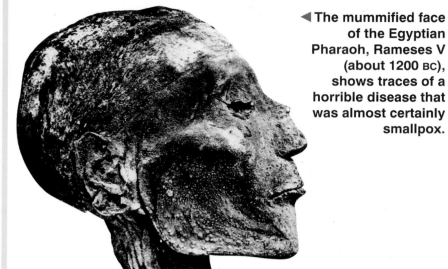

◀ **The mummified face of the Egyptian Pharaoh, Rameses V (about 1200 BC), shows traces of a horrible disease that was almost certainly smallpox.**

Vein A blood vessel that carries blood back to the heart.

Virus A micro-organism, much smaller than a bacterium, that reproduces itself inside the cells of the organism it invades and often causes disease.

X-rays Light-like radiation, but with a shorter wavelength and invisible to the human eye. X-rays can pass through watery body tissue but are absorbed by bones and other denser material. This enables doctors to obtain photographs of internal parts of their patients.

 # GOING FURTHER

Books The Health Education Council publishes a range of information books and leaflets on healthy living and the prevention of disease. Your local library or bookshop will also have a wide range of books on health and medicine. Here are some titles to look out for:
Eyewitness Science Guides: How the Body Works by Steve Parker, Dorling Kindersley 1994
The Body Atlas by Guiliano Fornari and Steve Parker, Dorling Kindersley 1993
Timelines: Medicine by Kathryn Senior, Watts 1993
X-Ray Picture Books: Your Body by Kathryn Senior, Watts 1993
Magazines Special interest magazines on health

matters are available from newsagents. Specialist magazines, such as *New Scientist*, contain items on the latest developments in medical research.
Places to visit In Britain, the Natural History Museum in London has a permanent exhibition on the Human Body. The Pharmaceutical Society's Museum in London, the Museum of the Royal College of Surgeons in Edinburgh and the Museum of the History of Science in Oxford all contain material relating to medicine and are worth visiting.
CD-ROM The following are worth considering:
Bodyworks 3.0, Guildsoft, Telephone 01752 89 5100
The Ultimate Human Body, Dorling Kindersley Multimedia 1994.

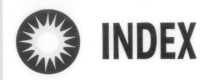

INDEX